# So You Wanna Live Forever?

*Twenty Tips to Be Forever Twenty-one*

~

Adam Dave, M.D.

# ONE

When I was a boy, I used to want to be six feet tall. I wanted this so badly that I devoted an entire summer, the summer of my 16th year, to the business of growing taller.

Every day I'd eat my vegetables (for the vitamins and the calories), drink my milk (for the calcium), and hang upside down on my parents' back swing. I refused to let my friends lure me into the gym at an age when your bench press pretty much defined your masculinity. But I was told weights "stunted growth," and so I lifted nothing heavier than my next glass of milk.

I was worried that like my mother and father, who had reached their adult heights (5'4 and 5'9, respectively) in their early teens, I had topped out. In fact, no one in my family on either side had managed to break the six-foot barrier. My half-brother, Jason, is 6'1", but he doesn't count, I'd later come to realize, because he had his mother's genes, and she had tall brothers.

I didn't think of this at the time, because I didn't realize that height is largely a genetic trait. In fact, short of starving yourself, restricting the intake of certain nutrients, or surgically installing an extra vertebra, there is little you can do to influence your adult stature either way. Like hair or eye color, height is hereditary.

And though each day I'd visit the kitchen wall and mark my height in pencil, at the end of the summer the marking had failed to budge even a millimeter from where it had been the previous June. I was stuck at 5'9'1/2, and have remained there ever since. Barring vertebral fractures and postural indiscretions, which can only sever precious centimeters, I will likely remain this tall (or short) until the day I die, which if life span is anything like height, I could at least say lay far into the future.

You see, I may come from a family of short people, but many of them were long-lived. For instance, my great, great grandfather on my mother's side was said to be 115. We have pictures of him, at well over 100, sitting in the yard with two young boys, one around eight and another in his early teens. They were his *sons* (by his third wife; he had outlived the first two). His daughter, my great grandmother, lived to be 104. Because of these and other examples, I consoled myself with the belief that though I had been denied tallness, longevity was my birthright.

But this is not the case.

It turns out that your life span is nothing like your height. Consider that identical twins sharing all the same genes die more than 10 years apart, on average. This is because unlike height, longevity is influenced by diet and lifestyle and other factors like mood and mindset, which are to a considerable degree under an individual's control. In short, we are largely responsible for our old age, and our death.

But first, let's be clear about one thing: Nobody dies of old age.

We've all heard the term "death by natural causes," but this is also untrue. It is a euphemism for organ failure, which is in most cases the true killer. The organs most likely to fail are the heart, the brain, the kidneys, the lungs, and the liver.

Most organs can regenerate, meaning damage can be repaired. In some organs the process of regeneration can go on indefinitely. Meaning we don't have to get old. And by extension, we don't have to die.

But we do.

In fact, about 100,000 people die worldwide each day of "natural causes," or roughly 90 percent in the industrialized world. This means that for every person who dies of all causes other than aging added together – be it homicide, suicide, road accidents, AIDS, whatever - ten people die of the euphemistic "old age."

Today, man's maximum life span is about 120 years, fully-authenticated. (The Abkhazians of Russia are purported to live into their 150s routinely, but this has never been reliably documented.) Today our average life expectancy is around 75 years, and climbing. Cro-magnon man lived to be an average of 18. In ancient Egypt the life expectancy was around 25. In Europe in the 1400s it was 30. In 1900 it climbed to 48 in the United States. In 2002, the life expectancy in the US was 78, and it's even higher in some countries (for instance in Japan, where the average woman reaches her mid-eighties).

In the last hundred years we've added nearly thirty years to the average life expectancy in the industrialized world. The media celebrates this, neglecting to mention that today's average modern adult spends more than 10 percent of his or her life sick, a ten-fold increase from 100 years ago. Nearly half of all Americans over the age of eighty-five have Alzheimer's disease. The average person living in the industrialized world consumes more health-care resources in his or her last year of life than in an entire life up to that point. Here I am reminded of my grandfather, George Dave, who at the age of 78 spent three months in the hospital with a heart condition, had surgery, recovered, got out of the hospital only to be hit by a car and die shortly thereafter.

By 2025, the annual cost of managing chronic conditions in the United States will exceed a trillion dollars. But though modern medicine is equipped to extend the *quantity* of years, it is far less able to ensure their *quality*. The medical model is focused on illness rather than wellness. As a family physician friend of mine has said, medicine as practiced today is sick care rather than health care. And the modern elderly adult is extremely ill. Often he is hunched over, incoherent, and slow – rather than agile and mentally lucid, with a sense of humor and admirable physical health who enjoys tranquility, as was once written of the long-lived Vilcamba people of Peru.

Most people hit their physical peak between twenty and thirty and gradually decline after that. Running is regarded as one of the few sports in which the hindering effects of age on performance are minimized, and it is true that runners in their late 60s are often as fast as runners in their late teens. But what about the ages in between? Analyze some of the world's biggest marathons (New York, Boston, Chicago), and you'll see that the fastest times are logged by guys between the ages of 20 and 34, with very few exceptions. After that, the times fall off precipitously. Every 5 to 10 years beyond the mid 30s witnesses a decline in marathon finish times of 10 minutes or more.

And it's not only athletic performance that plummets with age. By the age of seventy, most have lost 60 percent of their maximal breathing capacity, 40 percent of their kidney and liver functions, 15 to 30 percent of their bone mass, and 30 percent of their strength. Not to mention dementia and other types of cognitive decline, which occur almost exclusively in the elderly.

It would seem from this that death and taxes are not the only unavoidables. Add to the list senescence, which is a fancy way of saying, you guessed it: old age.

Often it is the heart which usually breaks down long before the rest of the body, and often very prematurely. (Which brings to mind my other grandfather, who had three heart attacks by the age of 52, the third of which did him in.) If you are a woman in North America, you have nearly a 50 percent chance of dying from heart disease – ten times your risk of dying from breast cancer. By contrast, Okinawans (a region of Japan) have only a fifth as many heart attacks as North Americans. In fact, Okinawa boasts more centenarians than any other place on earth. But by Biblical standards, even the Japanese could be said to die prematurely. Methusaleh lived to see nearly 1,000.

But you may not take the Bible literally, or see Adam, who lived to be 930, or even Abraham, who came 20 generations after Adam and lived to be 175, as historical figures. Like the character in Nacho Libre, you may believe in science. And in science there exists what is called the 2 billion heartbeat hypothesis. Believers (and there are many) see the heart rate as a determinant of lifespan. According to this hypothesis, the slower your heart rate, the longer you can expect to live. An extremely physically fit person with a rate of 45 beats per minute should therefore live 110 years.

But while a faster heart rate is indeed a marker for a shorter life expectancy, it is disputed whether there is any truth to the notion that the heart has a finite number of beats after which it is fated to expire. Nevertheless there is another theory with which to contend: namely, that most living species have an upper limit on the number of times their cells can divide. For humans, this is called the Hayflick limit. Scientists are hard at work finding ways to skirt this cellular expiration date, whether real or imaginary, and their research involves things like telomeres and intracellular and extracellular aggregates, which we shall touch on.

What kills us now? Of the top ten killers - heart disease, cancer, lower respiratory tract disease, stroke, accidents, Alzheimer's, diabetes, renal disease, pneumonia, suicide – most are degenerative, progressive diseases which taken together account for about 90 percent of the deaths in society. (The other 10 percent coming from medical errors, so called iatrogenic causes or physician-induced deaths, a product of our flawed medical system.) And most are more or less preventable.

Preventable. This includes cancer. Never mind that 1 in 2 people will be diagnosed with cancer at some point in life. It is estimated that in the United States over 1,500,000 men and women will be diagnosed with cancer in 2013. And nearly 600,000 men and women will die. That's more Americans than perished in World War I and World War II combined!!! (520,000)

But this staggering statistic is not true for other parts of the world. In Okinawa for instance, death rates from breast cancer are only 15% of what they are in America; deaths from other reproductive cancers, as well as colon cancer, are unheard of compared to the US, where prostate cancer is the second leading cause of death from cancer in men. More supercentenarians (people who live to be 110 and beyond) hail from Okinawa than anyplace else in the world. And they are healthy for most of their lives: The vast majority of those who make it to age 100 have been free of major diseases into their nineties, writes John Robbins in his wonderful book Healthy at 100.

(But this seeming immunity to cancer and heart disease seen in the Okinawans is not genetic: When they move to places where these diseases are prevalent, they are just as likely to suffer a heart attack or get cancer as the next person.)

And it's not just the Okinawans. The Hunza of Pakistan do not get cancer or diabetes. They live well past the century mark with no heart disease or high blood pressure. Which is no surprise, if you believe Dr. Norman Shealy, neurosurgeon, psychologist, and father of holistic medicine, who has compiled a list of healthy habits which can easily extend the average life expectancy from the world's current average of 77 years to at least 100. These include not smoking (which adds 6 years to your life), maintaining a healthy body weight (tack on another 6 years), abstaining from street drugs (1.5 years), drinking no more than one alcoholic drink per day, on average (3 years), and exercising a minimum of 7 hours per week (6 years). If you are a woman, notes Shealy, you can add another 2.6 years to your life expectancy. Married men can add 2.6 additional years, though marriage does not confer any longevity benefits for women. The world's longest lived people naturally abide by Dr. Shealy's healthy habits. They are active, lean, and avoid drugs and tobacco, while drinking in moderation if at all. And as we've said many of them live to see 100, even 120, after which they typically experience a rapid terminal decline.

But the point is, they do die, and no later than 120 years young.

If the incidence of heart disease and cancer and other Western killers is so low among the world's longest-lived people, then what are they dying of? In other words, what do we need to address if we are to catapult beyond the 120-year barrier and do so in the peak of vibrancy?

A theoretical physicist once wrote that in biology nothing has been discovered that indicates the inevitability of death, that it is only a matter of time before this terrible universal disease (aging, death) will be cured.

It is estimated that eliminating 50 percent of medically preventable conditions would extend human life expectancy to over 150 years. By preventing 99 percent of medical problems, we'd routinely live to be over one thousand years. In short, we'd all be Methusalehs!

Preventing preventable diseases should be pretty simple, shouldn't it? But then why has science felt the need to devise such fancy technologies in the battle against aging? Things like therapeutic cloning of human cells; downloading the brain onto computers; replacement of worn-out organs with android parts; respirocytes, nanobots, computerized neural implants, and foglets. Ray Kurzweil, futurist author of The Singularity, believes that the history of evolution can be divided into six epochs. We are currently in Epoch 5, which Kurzweil calls the Merger of Technology and Human Intelligence. He predicts a near future in which we essentially become computers, and they us.

While this may or may not happen (though it certainly makes for good science fiction), anyone who has suffered a flat tire or broken plumbing or had their computer crash on them knows that relying on technology can set a person up to be frustrated and even helpless. We must first focus on the things that are under our control before we look to the current medical model to provide a gateway into immortality because, sadly, the nation's health care system, irrational, uncoordinated, and inefficient as it is, spends more than two-thirds of every dollar treating preventable chronic diseases in order to slightly delay the inevitable.

Which, whether it has to be or not, is death.

For most, death is a tragedy. Unless you've lived a long and full life or are suffering a condition so distressing as to make life unbearable, it is hard to greet your personal end of days with anything approaching calm acceptance, and even after living a great many number of glorious years, or a painfully-ridden few, leaving the world behind is no walk in the park. Depending on your religious views, death may or may not be synonymous with the cessation of existence, *but it certainly implies a major change!*

A person, like a snowflake, is a unique expression never before seen and never to be repeated, and irretrievably lost when he or she dies. That, at least, is the case today, since we do not yet have the means to access and back up the intricate neural patterns accumulated in the brain over the course of a lifetime. When a loved one passes away, we truly lose a part of ourselves, since we no longer use the part of our brain wired to interact with that person.

My brother Justin died at the age of 22. Shortly after he left this earth, my father, who had read all sorts of books and visited all sorts of healers during Justin's six-month bout with terminal hip cancer, became convinced that we could extend the lifespan indefinitely (never mind that Justin had just passed away – his way of living, replete with alcohol, cigarettes, animal products, and recreational drugs, was a recipe for early demise, especially when coupled with the heart condition with which he was born). When my dad proposed the prospect of living forever, my response was, "Why in God's name would anyone want to live longer than we already do?" Sure, I was a bit disenchanted. My brother was gone and my parents were going through a divorce, and though I was in the full bloom of health with a whole life ahead of me, my philosophy could be summed up by the words of Moses (who by the way lived to be 120): "The days of our lives are seventy years; and if by reason of strength they are eighty years, yet their boast is only labor and sorrow; for it is soon cut off, and we fly away."

My "why bother?" attitude needed an adjustment, and I would come to find that as far as living to a ripe old age is concerned, attitude is everything, for longevity is just as much spiritual as it is physical, perhaps more, and self-confidence counts. Self-confidence happens to be precisely what my brother Justin lacked.

After that conversation with dad, I forgot about death, and for fifteen years drank deeply of the cup of youth. I wrote novels and screenplays, travelled, drank a lot of beer, and earned my medical degree. Then my mother - who had been diagnosed with breast cancer just prior to her 50th birthday, was treated and went into remission - relapsed in 2010, at the age of 65. This got me once again to start thinking about mortality, but not my own. I didn't start thinking about my own death until I turned 40. At around this time things started happening that made me question my invincibility. Things like: A cracked rib while giving a friend a chiropractic adjustment (I am not a chiropractor and shouldn't have tried the maneuver); a metatarsal stress fracture as a result of overzealous running; a chipped tooth resulting from overly vigorous flossing. Hair loss on my legs in a sock-like distribution, which can be an early sign of heart disease, and despite a vigorous workout regimen and vegan diet! Hangovers that happened two drinks too soon. Wrinkles around the eyes and sun spots made it increasingly more of a downer to regard myself in the mirror, especially since I reside in tinsel town, where the emphasis on physical appearance is so great, and where ever larger swaths of the population, at an ever earlier age, are undergoing cosmetic procedures to preserve the semblance of youth. I know that beauty is not merely skin deep, but this provided me with little consolation, as beneath my integument my body felt the way my tired eyes looked. Vague and sometimes sharp, shooting pains, especially in the joints, started paying me a visit and staying for longer and longer periods of time, pains that have been around for so long now I am becoming less and less optimistic that they'll ever go away.

As it became increasingly clear that my body was breaking down (or aging, if you like, but I refused to equate the two terms) I was left wondering what good a long life was if the body was ill-equipped to fully enjoy it, and for that matter growing ever less equipped as the days went by.

I complained to my mother, who said I may not feel like running marathons into my 80s, that my priorities would likely change with advancing age, that I'd become more involved in other things (kids, grandkids, volunteer work). But what if I wanted to continue to run marathons but was physically unable to do so any longer?

A defining feature of unhappiness is being unable to do what one wishes to do. Forever may or may not come, but what about today? Before we go into whether it's possible to live forever, we must first ask whether we'd want to even try, and even before that we need to consider why we age, and why we die.

TWO

Remember when I said your life span was not hereditary? Well, some of it is. Evidence from the human genome project indicates that just a few hundred genes out of the tens of thousands hidden in our DNA are involved in the aging process. But it is not so much genes as *epi*genes that are the real factors in longevity. Epigenes are molecules not part of our DNA but which are responsible for the activity of genes and their expression. They are influenced by lifestyle factors including diet. For example, eating excessively and becoming obese can alter these epigenes, which influences the way genes are expressed, and these changes are inheritable, so that you pass to your kids a tendency to gain weight. And diet is not the only area of life which can manipulate the expression of genes involved in the aging process. Meditation does as well. So does exercise. Or, if you like multitasking, meditating while exercising, which we'll discuss.

A key factor in aging is something known as a telomere. Telomeres are repeating segments of DNA found at the end of chromosomes. Each time a cell reproduces, one segment drops off. Telomeres therefore get shorter each year, from birth to death, at a constant rate that averages 1%

a year. They are a marker for aging; the older the person, the shorter their telomeres. Once a cell has reproduced to the point that it reaches a critical telomere length, that cell is no longer able to divide and so it dies. The telomeres of cancer cells do not shorten, because cancer is equipped with the enzyme telomerase, which lengthens telomere segments. It is believed that if we could reverse this process, in other words prevent telomeres from shortening or even increase their length, we could get normal cells to survive indefinitely, just as cancer cells do. And in fact this has shown to be the case in studies. Bad lifestyle habits accelerate the process of telomere shortening, and good ones slow it down slightly. Some scientists believe the process can be reversed in human beings, in part with the help of a healthy diet and exercise routine.

One such scientist is Aubrey DeGrey, a pioneer in the field of anti-aging research. DeGrey has developed his own unique views on our subject. Focusing on molecular damage as the chief cause of aging, he has developed a list of the cellular events leading to such damage. His list includes:

One – mutations in the chromosomes

Two – glycation, the warping of proteins by glucose commonly seen in diabetes and insulin resistance (conditions more common as we grow older)

Three – extracellular aggregates, the various kinds of junk that accumulate outside the cell, including beta-amyloid and transthyretin.

Four – intracellular aggregates, for example lipofuscin pigments, which build up within the cell. Lipofuscin is what remains of unsuccessfully degraded mitochondria, damaged by the effects of free radicals.

DeGrey believes that the failure to dispose of specific waste products is at the root of the most terrible diseases that accompany aging: atherosclerosis, macular degeneration, and neurodegenerative diseases such as Alzheimer's. Chalk it up to bad housecleaning.

Five – cellular senescence, the aging of individual cells, which puts them into a state of arrested growth and causes them to produce chemical signals dangerous to neighboring structures.

Six – depletion of the stem cell pools essential to healing and maintenance of tissue.

Seven – mutations in the mitochondria, the energy factories of the cell. Defective mitochondria generate more free radicals, which leads to aging.

DeGrey, who believes we can probably eliminate aging as a cause of death this century, believes that diet and exercise are a good start but fall short of the mark as far as extending the lifespan indefinitely. Instead he proposes very advanced, technologically-dependent ways of addressing the above problems, such as vaccines against amyloid plaque and stem cells cultured in the lab to be delivered as a rejuvenating cellular therapy.

But the trick about laboratory work, the catch that DeGrey himself admits, is the butterfly effect:

tinker with one mechanism and you get unpredictable ramifications on other mechanisms. For example, free radicals cause oxidative stress and damage over time. If you flood the system with antioxidants to defend against free radicals, you could in fact provide cancer cells with a defense against the powerful chemotherapeutic drugs designed to kill them.

But whether or not we employ science in our fight for forever, first it is key to address people's attitudes to aging. In what is called the pro-aging trance, people are convinced that getting older is a part of life, that at certain points they will experience the all-too-common symptoms of old age: aches, pains, and loss of function. Or to paraphrase Billy Crystal in the movie <u>City Slickers</u>, losing hair where you want it and growing hair where you don't. If a common reaction to suggesting even a modest postponement of aging is to cry out against the woes of overpopulation and resource depletion, what happens when you try telling someone that aging as a cause of infirmity and death can be eliminated forever? You are likely to be rewarded with a black eye!

In order to break the trance we must first face the facts. Aging is a disease, a downward spiral, and once it starts it's hard to stop. The more we age, the less able our body is to stop us from aging, so we age faster and faster. So it's to be expected that the late stages of aging, the organ diseases, go faster than the earlier stages, and if you've ever visited the ICU, you've witnessed the rapid decline that patients there undergo.

Does it have to be this way? I am reminded of a friend of the family who told me when I got my first car, "Just take it in regularly for an oil change and lube, and it will run forever." The question we must answer is whether the same or similar can be said about the human vehicle.

Science would argue yes. The human body is in a constant state of renewal. The entire human skeleton renews itself about every ten years. The regenerative capacity of the body is amazing, provided we give it what it needs (which can be as simple as fresh air, clean water, nutritious food, and regular movement), and simply stay out of its way.

Perhaps more important than the body in its influence on aging is the mind. Our emotions and behavior shape our brains as they stimulate the formation of neural pathways that either reinforce old patterns or initiate new ones. Most of your genes are engaged in cooperation with signals from the environment and are influenced by signals that don't come from the DNA but from proteins surrounding your genetic code, the aforementioned epigenes. Epigenetics studies the changes (often inheritable) in gene function that occur without a change in the DNA sequence, the sources that control gene expression from outside the DNA. It's the study of the signals that turn genes on and off. Some of those signals are chemical, others are electromagnetic. Some come from inside the body, while others are the body's response to signals from the outside environment.

These signals initiate stem cell differentiation and wound healing, and impact longevity.

In essence, your beliefs become your biology. Evidence suggests that the epigenetic signals that make one person youthful and energetic and another haggard and decrepit come from outside the gene, outside the cell, and sometimes outside the body. This is exciting news, if you're a person that likes control. DNA is not your destiny. You have much more control over the quality and quantity of your years than was ever before believed. With every feeling and thought, in every moment of your life, you are performing epigenetic engineering on your own cells, helping them regenerate and strengthen, or causing them to pale and die.

If you take nothing away from this book other than this, you will have learned something invaluable.

So, whether or not forever is in the cards for humans as a species, as an individual it will be worth your while to pay heed to the following pointers and you will go far to ensure that your days, if not unnumbered, will most certainly be unencumbered. That not only can you add to the *quantity* but also the *quality* of your years. Some are old hat, others may surprise you, all are honored by time and upheld by scientific evidence, so make them your friends.

## THREE

John Knowles, late president of the Rockefeller Foundation, famously said that 85 percent of all illness is a consequence of lifestyle choices. Included in his definition of an unhealthy lifestyle are things like the use of tobacco, street drugs, and excess alcohol; inactivity; and negative attitudes. We can add to this list poor dietary choices resulting in nutrient deficiencies and excessive caloric intake, and the direct consequence of a poor diet: namely, weight gain and/or increased body fat percentage.

Let's start with these and build from there.

**1. Don't smoke**

This is a no-brainer, so we'll be brief.

Smokers live over a decade shorter than nonsmokers.

Cigarette smoking is the leading cause of preventable death, accounting for more than 440,000 deaths, or one of every five deaths, in the US each year.

And yet nearly 50 million American adults continue to smoke cigarettes. Smokeless tobacco, cigars, and pipes also have deadly consequences, including lung, larynx, esophageal, and oral cancers.

The body has such powerful capacity for regeneration that if a lifelong smoker quits for 15 years his risk of diseases including heart disease, stroke, and yes, lung cancer, is as low as the nonsmoker's.

Take-home point: *If you don't smoke, don't start. If you do smoke, quit now.*

## 2. Drink in moderation, if at all

Alcohol has been around for millennia, and moderate consumption is not without possible health benefits. For example, if your blood pressure runs high, alcohol can help bring it down. If you have atherosclerotic plaques, alcohol can dilate the blood vessels to effectively enlarge their width and render you less susceptible to coronary events. But a little goes a long way. Each of the long-living cultures enjoys alcoholic beverages, but only in moderation. Too much alcohol can damage a variety of organs, including the brain, liver, even the heart which moderate drinking is said to protect.

You may be like many people who like to unwind with a cocktail or two. But alcohol's effects on the body are anything but relaxing. It is a potent neurotoxin, and it stimulates the liver which must work overtime in order to detoxify it, essentially by breaking it down in a two-step enzymatic process. And though alcohol can mitigate some of the ill effects of dietary indiscretions, it should be remembered that there are no advantages to consuming alcohol that are not matched/exceeded with abiding by a nutritious diet, our next topic.

Take-home point: *Moderate drinking is defined as one drink per day if you're a woman, two if you're a man. One drink is a 12-ounce bottle of 5% beer, a 5-ounce glass of 12% wine, or 1.5 ounces of 40% hard liquor.*

## 3. Eat unprocessed plant foods

It has been said that the incidence of cancer increases in direct proportion to the civilization of a people. Indeed the most common diseases of the civilized world – not only cancer but heart disease, diabetes, asthma, arthritis, and obesity – also called diseases of affluence, are rare among indigenous peoples whose diet consists of fresh, unprocessed foods, grown in their environment.

The world's longest-lived people are to a large degree without the wrinkles, gray hairs, baldness, and need for glasses which have come to define our contemporary notion of old age. Without exception they eat a raw or lightly-cooked, low-calorie, plant-based, whole-foods diet. (Such a diet, notes best-selling author Joel Fuhrman, M.D., has indeed been observed to restore the natural pigment to gray hair.) They derive the majority of their calories from carbohydrates (75%), with comparatively modest amounts of fat (15%) and protein (10%). In other words, they eat a high-carbohydrate diet consisting of about 2,000 calories per day, low by Western standards, and 99% of those calories are derived from plants.

Their diet is without exception naturally low in salt and without processed sugars. Incidence of obesity: zero.

The healthfulness of this lifestyle is corroborated by the leading scientific evidence, which tells us to choose predominantly plant-based foods including vegetables and fruits, legumes, and minimally processed starchy staple foods to prevent the majority of all cancers, cardiovascular diseases, and other forms of degenerative illness.

In 2005 the Journal of the American Medical Association published a study that compared four popular diets including Atkins and the Zone, and it was the plant-based high-complex-carbohydrate diet promoted by Dean Ornish, M.D. that most effectively led to weight loss, lower cholesterol, and increased insulin sensitivity. Complex carbs include fruits, vegetables, and beans.

The research of Dr. Roy Walford, father of the calorie restriction longevity movement, demonstrated the manifold benefits of the nutrient-dense, low-calorie diet enjoyed by indigenous centenarians. These benefits extend beyond the extension seen in both average and maximum life spans. Such a diet postpones the onset and decreases the frequency of age-related disease, maintains biomarkers at levels younger than chronological age, keeps sexual potency at its peak, while sustaining the ability to engage in sports into advanced age and delaying deterioration of the brain. Walford included animal products in his calorically-restricted diet.

Perhaps had he shunned them in favor of plants, he'd have lived beyond age 79. (Here we are reminded of the passage from the book The Coming Race, which spoke of a race of people who "degraded their rank and shortened their lives by eating the flesh of animals.")

It is no longer necessary to even include minimal amounts of animal protein in the diet. It used to be that diets shunning seafood and dairy risked a deficit in nutrients including vitamin B-12 and omega-3 fatty acids, but nutritional yeast and flaxseeds are now popular vegan choices, and if nutrient deficiencies are a concern there is always the trusty multivitamin.  Flax is far superior to fish as the go-to source of omega fats, containing as it does as much as 800 times more lignans (anti-oxidants) than any other food. Due to the sorry state of our oceans even fish caught in the wild likely contains dangerous levels of heavy metals and other harmful substances. And forget about farmed fish, which accounts for 90 percent of fish on the market. Farmed fish is high in pcbs, dioxins, insecticides, and mercury.

Many health risks lurk in animal foods. Heme iron, the type of iron present in meat, speeds the aging process.

Processed foods, especially those high in sugar, are also a concern. Food divorced from the water and fiber present in the whole state, as is found with sugary soft-drinks and candies, plays havoc with blood sugar, which increases the amounts of AGEs, advanced glycation end-products. Like heme iron, AGEs cause oxidative stress and contributes to aging and disease. (Don't substitute sugar for sweeteners such as aspartame and think you're serving your health, as aspartame is a known poison.)

And cooking food (particularly meat) until it blackens as is often the case with grilled meats, increases levels of heterocyclic amines, which are cancer-causing substances. Cooking at high temperature without water – as in baking, broiling, grilling, roasting and frying at high temperatures - also causes AGEs to form. These toxic byproducts are therefore found in high concentrations in baked goods, meat, even roasted coffee. AGEs cause inflammation, which prevents your body from responding to insulin and sets you up for diabetes.

The temperature of foods cooked with water can never exceed 212 degrees, and water-based cooking methods allow water to combine with the sugars which prevents the sugars from attaching to proteins and fats. Examples of cooking with water include boiling, steaming, and sautéing in water or broth. The higher the temperature, the more of these sugar-fat and sugar-protein complexes appear in the food.

Foods containing GMO (genetically-modified organisms) should also be avoided as they increase the ageing process. The top GMO foods are soy, canola, and corn. Buy these and as many other foods as you can organic, which will also go far in protecting you from exposure to harmful pesticides and fertilizers found in most food items, including fruits and vegetables. The dirty dozen (most contaminated fruits and vegetables) are peaches, apples, sweet bell peppers, celery, nectarines, strawberries, cherries, pears, imported grapes, spinach, lettuce, and potatoes.

Take-home point: *Eat predominantly plant-foods in their raw and lightly-cooked state. Emphasize fruits, vegetables, starchy staples (beans, potatoes, bananas) and some healthy fats in the form of avocados, olives, and some seeds.*

## 4. Drink water

Everyone knows water is good for you, but exactly how good is it, and what benefits can it offer in terms of longevity?

First, consider that you are made up of mostly water, 70 percent or more. If you weigh 150 pounds, that's over 100 pounds. Water serves a variety of essential physiological functions. It is the main solvent for all foods, vitamins, and minerals. It is used to transport oxygen and nutrients to the cells and clear toxic waste to the liver and kidneys for disposal. It lubricates joint spaces. It even generates electrical and magnetic energy inside the cells.

According to Dr. F. Batmanghelidj, M.D., author of the book <u>Your Body's Many Cries for Water</u>, good ole H20 provides a number of additional benefits, some of them pretty far out. The good doctor states that water stimulates the enzymes that burn fat and permanently reduce weight, "causing you to lose 30-50 pounds without any effort," makes your brain work like an atomic clock, restores your enthusiasm, and fills you with the joys of life, in addition to being an anticancer medication, bolstering the immune system, and preventing/curing a wide variety of conditions including depression, asthma, and high blood pressure. Batmanghelidj states that water can even prevent autoimmune disease, memory loss, and cure addictions. Some pretty outlandish claims, these. But are they any more outlandish than the belief (held by patients, physicians, and pharmaceuticals) that depression can be cured with a pill? One would think it easier, less expensive, and far more natural to try water first.

The recommendations are to ingest at least two quarts (8 cups) of water and some salt every day to compensate for the natural losses in urine, respiration, and perspiration. Added to the two quarts present in food, this comes to a gallon per day. This is to unburden the kidneys, which must work to concentrate urine in the setting of dehydration, and to properly hydrate the skin and soften stool. A rough rule of thumb is to drink one half an ounce for every pound of bodyweight. That's 75 ounces (just over 9 cups) if you weigh 150 pounds. Drink at least two glasses of water on awakening, one or two glasses half an hour before each major meal, and another one or two glasses a couple hours after eating. The latter helps empty the stomach of residual food and prevents the false sensation of hunger which some may feel between meals. And of course, drink water regularly throughout the day to avoid thirst. Don't wait until you are thirsty, as the popular saying goes: Thirst is actually a sign that you are already dehydrated. And remember to drink water before any physical activity. A good rule of thumb is to drink at least sixteen ounces (2 cups) for each 30 minutes you plan to exercise, more when exercising in hot weather.

What does the science have to say about the effect of water on performance? A lot, it turns out. A study from the University of Arkansas shows that a mild one percent dehydration (equivalent to 1.5 pounds of body weight, or 1.5 pints of fluid) has a negative impact on athletic ability. Dehydration was found to slow down competitive bicycle racers by a mile per hour, reduce power to pedal, raise stomach temperature, and lower sweat sensitivity that controls body temperature. It also increases perceived exertion, meaning riders could not tell that they rode more slowly when they were mildly dehydrated. How much is 1.5 pints of fluid? It can be lost in as short as one hour of exercising, even more rapidly on a hot day.

Doctors often use heart rate as an indicator of fluid status, because your heart beats faster as your blood volume diminishes. But after losing over a pound in body weight, the cyclists' heart rates remained the same, suggesting heart rate, like thirst, is an unreliable method for assessing hydration.

Take home point: *Drink at least two quarts of nonchlorinated water daily, more if you exercise. You are adequately hydrated if you urinate at least every two or three hours, and your urine is clear or light yellow.*

## 5. Say NO to Drugs

This goes for prescriptions as well as for illicit substances. No aspect of the American medical system is more flawed than the drug industry, notes Dr. Norman Shealy in his book <u>Life Beyond 100</u>. Deaths from prescription drug use in the United States are now over 110,000 per year. Prescribed substances cause over twice the number of deaths as street drugs, and nearly six times as many deaths as over-the-counter drugs. Drug-related illness, disability, and death is a huge problem in the medical system, and more deaths likely arise from taking medication than lives are saved by pills.

You'd never know this, judging from the prevalence of prescriptive medications. Nearly 70 percent of Americans are on at least one prescription drug, and more than half receive at least two prescriptions. Twenty percent of US patients are on five or more meds. This does not include over-the-counter remedies such as Tylenol and aspirin, which are not without health risks, among them liver and kidney disorders, stomach ulcers, and excessive bleeding. Antibiotics, antidepressants and painkiller opioids are the most commonly prescribed drugs. One in four middle-aged women is on an anti-depressant, a drug taken by over 10 percent of the population, making drugs like Zoloft, Prozac, and Paxil hugely popular, despite the fact that these drugs have been shown to be, in many cases, virtually useless. While only minimally better than placebo (water pill), they carry great risks, including mood or behavior changes, anxiety, panic attacks, trouble sleeping, impulsivity, irritability, agitation, hostility, aggression, restlessness, hyperactivity, increased depression, and suicidal thoughts. Physical symptoms attending antidepressant use include insomnia, skin rashes, headaches, joint and muscle pain, stomach upset, nausea, or diarrhea muscle spasms, and diminished sexual appetite.

We haven't mentioned the inactive ingredients used as fillers and coatings for drugs. Take Zoloft, for instance. The active ingredient is the antidepressant sertraline, a selective serotonin reuptake inhibitor (SSRI). But the drug also contains a list of inactive ingredients including dibasic calcium phosphate dihydrate, D & C Yellow #10 aluminum lake, FD & C Blue #1 aluminum lake, FD & C Red #40 aluminum lake, FD & C Blue #2 aluminum lake, hydroxypropyl cellulose, hypromellose, magnesium stearate, microcrystalline cellulose, polyethylene glycol, polysorbate 80, sodium starch glycolate, synthetic yellow iron oxide, and titanium dioxide.

It's not only antidepressants that are well-nigh ineffective in treating diseases when compared to lifestyle choices. Take the cholesterol-lowering statin drug Lipitor. Eating a healthy diet is three times more effective for preventing a recurrent heart attack, and without the side effect profile that includes muscle pain, liver damage, nausea and diarrhea.

Take-home point: *If you don't use drugs, don't start. If you do, see about clearing out your medicine cabinet, with a health-care professional's approval, of course.*

## 6. Be lean

Obesity contributes more to chronic illness and healthcare costs than does smoking. To put a positive spin on it, we can say that superior health is defined by an exceptionally long and disease-free life, and a large body of scientific evidence shows that people with superior health are slim. Why is this?

Slim people generally have lower body fat, particularly visceral fat. Visceral fat is most visible around your middle, contributing to what is often called an apple-shaped body. It clumps around major internal organs like the liver and kidneys. In contrast to subcutaneous fat (which is located just under the skin and tends to accumulate in the hips and thighs, contributing to the classic "pear" shape), visceral fat is not just inert storage space. Rather, it is metabolically active, dynamic tissue. It secretes and responds to a variety of hormones and other signaling molecules.

Fat contains a mixture of different cell types, including connective tissue, nerves, and blood vessels, as well as immune cells such as macrophages. Indeed, adipocytes (fat cells) are derived from the same cell line as macrophages, and they secrete many of the same immune-system-stimulating, pro-inflammatory molecules called cytokines, among them tumor necrosis factor alpha, as well as interleukins.

As fat builds up (and it tends to do this as you get older), fat cells dump more inflammatory mediators into the system. Scientists have been trying to develop drugs to do encourage the body to burn off excess visceral fat, but there does not seem to be a magic pill. Experiments with the appetite-regulating hormone leptin have shown it to be ineffective as a weight loss treatment, and while amphetamines produce results, their side effects and addictiveness far outweigh the benefits of rapid weight loss.

Excess body fat also increases the body's resistance to insulin. (Insulin regulates the amount of sugar in your blood. Insulin resistance causes sugar to build up in the blood and creates AGEs, which contribute to aging.) In fact, when you compare people of different ages, the difference in insulin response between young and old disappears when you account for the difference in visceral fat. Young people have less visceral fat and are more responsive to insulin, which keeps their blood sugar at a normal level, while older people tend to have more visceral fat and are insulin-resistant. Are older people doomed to age by forming AGEs? Not necessarily. When we look at age-related loss of muscle and increase in fat, we find that it is not a function of years lived but of loss of activity. In other words, people tend to become more sedentary with age, which leads to the changes in body composition (more fat, less muscle) and it is this change that causes insulin resistance and inflammation. And the loss of muscle due to inactivity encourages more inactivity. A use it or lose it vicious cycle we will explore shortly.

The good news is that visceral fat is the first thing to go when your caloric needs aren't met, so weight loss as a result of calorie reduction or increased exercise, or a combination of both, significantly improves insulin resistance and reduces inflammation rather quickly.

Diet and exercise work wonders.

Why is too much inflammation bad? While some inflammation serves a healthful purpose – to fight infection and heal wounds, for example - the inflammatory cascade, if allowed to surge out of control, can wreak havoc on your body. It attacks your joints to cause arthritis, your kidneys to cause kidney failure, your heart to cause a heart attack, and your pancreas to cause diabetes.

Optimal weight for most people can be calculated by taking 100 and adding 4 or 5 pounds for every one inch of height above 5 feet. A 5'10" male should weight 150 lbs and a 5'4" female about 116. To make sure your visceral fat levels are low, measure you waist and hip circumferences and determine your waist to hip ratio using any of a number of online resources.

Take-home point: *Lose the belly flab, first by restricting sources of trans fatty acids (found in fried foods and in hydrogenated vegetable oils) and favoring a whole foods, plant-based diet rich in a variety of fruits, vegetables, legumes, and seeds, and combining this* diet-style *with lots of physical activity, which happens to be our next topic.*

## 7. Exercise, in novel ways, preferably uphill

As people in the modern world get up there in years, they experience a predictable set of changes. They lose muscle mass and consequently become weaker. Their metabolism slows down. They lose aerobic capacity. Blood pressure and blood sugar rise, cholesterol levels worsen, bone density decreases, as does tolerance to cold weather.

Is it inevitable that as you age your strength diminishes, your reflexes slow, your eyesight deteriorates, and your physical coordination plummets? "Disuse syndrome" a term coined by marathoner and medical doctor Walter Bortz, describes how a lack of physical activity can destroy health and lead to rapid premature aging.

Scientists now use the pattern of impairment described above as a measure of biological aging, and they refer to blood pressure, blood sugar, and the like, as biomarkers. Studies at the Human Nutrition Research Center on Aging at Tufts University have shown that age-related changes associated with these biomarkers, far from being inevitable, can in fact be prevented and even reversed.

The average American loses over 5 pounds of muscle with each decade starting in his twenties, and the rate of muscle loss accelerates after the age forty-five. If you're a healthy male around the age of twenty-five, you probably have under 20 percent body fat. By the time you are sixty-five, if you are like most Americans, you will have nearly 40 percent body fat. But with regular vigorous physical activity, muscle strength and size can be maintained and even increased at virtually any age.

In the anti-aging community, human growth hormone, or hGH, is touted as a rejuvenator. It is very expensive and brings with it potential health risks. Regular exercise produces the same beneficial changes in the body as human growth hormone – increased muscle mass, decreased body fat, and stronger bones – but without the side effects seen with supplemental hGH.

Because muscle is highly metabolic (burns a lot of calories, even at rest), the higher the ratio of muscle to fat, the higher the metabolic rate. Increasing your muscle-to-fat ratio through vigorous exercise increases your aerobic capacity and stimulates the production of a rich network of capillaries, which improves circulation and maintains a steady supply of oxygen and nutrient-rich blood.

This all goes to show that much of the so-called age-related physical decline stems not from age but from simple lack of use. Our ancestors were able to run for miles well into their old age because their daily life revolved around physical exertion. When nomads left Africa about 60,000 years ago, they are said to have walked ten miles a day, and many indigenous peoples maintain this level of physical activity. But building exercise into the routines of daily life can be difficult in a society such as ours, a society so geared to being sedentary. Setting aside an hour or so each day for vigorous activity – preferably the morning for cardiovascular fitness, and the evening for strength training – just as you do for meals, chores, or watching TV, seems to work best for most people.

It is interesting to note that the world's longest-lived populations tend to be mountain dwellers. With the exception of Okinawa, they reside thousands of feet above sea level, where the air is thin and pure, and the terrain ideal for uphill exercise. Moving against gravity in rarified air means their hearts and lungs get a better workout on a daily basis, and negotiating rugged terrain is great for coordination and quick reflexes. But living at or near sea level can offer the same benefits provided you maintain a high level of activity, and it helps if you are able to locate a steep hill or flight of stairs nearby to walk or run up a few times.

The benefits of exercise go beyond the physical. Running and other forms of voluntary exercise are also associated with long-term improvements in mental function. Exercise is the single best thing you can do to slow the cognitive decline that accompanies normal aging, and it has a dramatic antidepressive effect, blunting the brain's response to physical and emotional stress. And the runner's high is a real phenomenon. Physical activity enhances memory and learning capacity, in addition to boosting attention and improving multi-tasking and decision making abilities, likely due to an increase in oxygen flow and neurotransmitter release. Researchers at Germany's University of Bonn scanned the brains of subjects after they had completed a two-hour run and found that levels of opioids (so-called feel good hormones) had risen significantly. Exercise also increases the levels of endocannabinoids, the brain's natural cannabis-like molecules, in the bloodstream. We are reminded of a study in which participants' death rates fell in proportion to the number of calories they burned each week, which supports the notion that more activity leads to greater longevity. In a study published in the European Heart Journal, researchers found that French Tour de France cyclists live six years longer than other Frenchmen. The bicycle racers included in the study had a 41 percent lower death rate than the general population. They also suffered far fewer cancers, heart attacks or lung diseases.

Exercise also increases the number of dopamine receptors in the brain. Dopamine is a reward chemical largely responsible for the euphoria experienced with drugs such as methamphetamine and cocaine. How to increase dopamine even further? Exercise in novel ways. Novel ways can mean a new activity, or a unique version of a conventional one. A personal favorite is to run barefoot. Even if you're not an attention-seeker, the looks and comments you get from running without shoes is sure to spur you forward at faster speeds, whether you are running a race or recreationally.

Exercise also increases one's VO2 max, an indicator of fitness and also, it so happens, a marker for longevity. Moreover, because working out generates free radicals, the body responds by increasing production of anti-oxidants, which goes on long after you stop training.

There is excellent evidence that exercise early in the morning – before breakfast – has greater benefit on caloric expenditures throughout the day than exercise at the end of the day, but however you choose to do it, being physically active is a healthy and inexpensive way to get high naturally and increase both the quality and quantity of your years.

Take-home point: *Get at least three hours weekly of moderate physical activity with a goal of seven to fourteen hours.*

## 8. Don't sit

The average person sits 64 hours per week, or 9 hours a day. And this does not include the 7 or 8 hours of nightly sleep (which puts the total time spent on your back or backside at closer to 17 hours per day, which is more than 2/3s of the time). Even those who engage in regular exercise are very sedentary when not training, either because of increased fatigue after a workout, or from a feeling of complacency.

Inactivity can promote a variety of potentially serious blood abnormalities such as lower blood plasma volume (allowing blood to sludge), higher hematocrit (concentration of hemoglobin), in addition to higher plasma fibrinogen, elevated blood viscosity, increased platelet aggregation, and diminished fibrinolysis, all of which make the blood more prone to clot and set the stage for heart attacks and strokes. Women increase their risk for diabetes with every 2 hours they sit, and men who spend 6 hours sitting down are more likely to die of heart disease or diabetes than men who sit for half as long.

Sitting is also associated with psychiatric conditions including panic disorder, hypochondriasis, depression, and phobias. Which is why experts are calling it the "sitting disease" and comparing it to smoking, which is bad for you no matter how much exercise you get and kale you eat.

What's so bad about sitting? A lot, it turns out. When you sit for prolonged periods (call it 20 minutes or more), blood pools in your lower extremities, reducing the flow to your brain of important chemicals, including those involved in mood. Sitting also turns off an important gene that prevents blood clotting and inflammation. What's more, the static position - back hunched, hips and knees flexed, head bent - is a postural nightmare that puts excessive stress on many major muscle groups, including your hip flexors, causes muscle imbalances in the glutes, hamstrings, and iliotibial band, and increases laxity in the ligaments of the spine, which can set you up for back pain.

We weren't meant to sit as long as we do, but society seems structured around the fat ass. Don't let that be you.

Take-home point: *If you must sit for long periods, make an effort every 20 minutes to stand up for at least a minute. But don't just stand there! Prolonged standing strains the legs and feet and is of no benefit to your circulation. The trick is to move. Walk around, do some squats or calf raises, do a hand stand. Even lying on the floor beside your desk will help to move blood back to your heart and head and straighten and align your spine.*

## 9. Sleep/Nap

Sleep is rarely mentioned as a major contributor to health and longevity. Today we average half as much sleep (five hours) compared to the 1700s, and yet we live much longer, but does lack of sleep negatively impact performance? Yes, says the science. Sleep deprivation impairs attention, working memory, long-term memory, and decision-making. And new research suggests that sleep deprivation can slow glucose metabolism by 30 to 40 percent and increase levels of the stress hormone cortisol. Even short-term sleep deprivation, such as not getting adequate sleep for even a few nights, can lead to weight gain and immune dysfunction. In fact, too little sleep can be as harmful to your health as a sedentary lifestyle.

So how much is enough sleep? If you ask ten different people, even ten different high achievers, how much shut-eye they get each night, you are likely to get ten different answers. Consider the old Einstein versus Edison argument. Thomas

Edison, on the one hand, claimed sleep to be a waste of time (he opted for naps), while Albert Einstein, on the other hand, acknowledged that he needed ten hours of nightly shut-eye for optimal performance.

What about the rest of us? For most individuals, peak alertness during the day occurs when they have slept between eight and nine hours at night, but if you exercise vigorously you may need as much as ten hours. Regular exercisers also tend to fall asleep in half the time it takes others.

Take-home point: *Sleep a minimum of seven nightly hours. If you have trouble falling asleep, make sure that your room is totally dark and completely quiet (if possible). If all else fails, eat a banana. If you need to catch up on sleep, take a nap. A short nap of 10-30 minutes helps improve mood, performance, and alertness and keeps you in good company: both Einstein and Edison are known to have valued an afternoon nap.*

## 10. Floss

Great grandma who lived to be 104 had dentures for as long as I can remember, and often she voiced the regret that she hadn't taken better care of her chompers. (Grandma loved candy.)

Tooth and gum disease goes beyond discolored teeth, discomfort, and bad breath, beyond even a root canal. The bacteria that flourish in an unhealthy mouth can harm the rest of the body and even lead to heart disease, diabetes and respiratory illness. This is such a significant issue that, in 2003, the Centers for Disease Control and Prevention (CDC) called for public health initiatives to promote oral health as an effective preventative measure for these and other life-threatening illnesses.

A protein known as C-reactive peptide, or CRP, is a measure of inflammation. Physicians draw a patient's CRP to monitor disease severity and response to treatment. It turns out that high levels of CRP are inversely correlated with longevity. In other words, the higher your CRP, the shorter your life. Periodontal disease is a leading cause of elevated CRP levels. Flossing can prevent/eliminate periodontal disease and normalize CRP levels, in turn leading to increased longevity.

Take-home point: *Take care of your teeth. Floss daily.*

## 11. Exfoliate

The skin is the largest organ in your body, and a principal organ of waste removal, via the sweat (although the chief function of sweat is temperature regulation). But if your pores are blocked by dead skin, the waste removal process may be hindered. Slough off dead skin regularly with a loofa, puff buff, body scrub, or body brush. Beach sand also works well. Scrub yourself from top to toe, but be careful not to overexfoliate, which can leave skin raw, red and vulnerable to bacteria.

Take-home point: *If lotions, creams and ointments fail to moisturize your skin, it is because the topmost layers are dead and need to be shed, so start scrubbing.*

## 12. Spend Time Outside

The benefits of sun exposure are many. Sun is an excellent source of vitamin D, needed for healthy bones, mood, and immune function. But being outdoors provides a host of goodness that goes beyond solar rays. You can hear the birds chirp or the squirrels wrestle for nuts. Lie in the grass, go barefoot on the beach, enjoy a sunset. These simple pleasures are free.

Take-home point: *Spend at least one hour daily outdoors.*

## 13. Help others/Be kind

In the world's healthiest and longest-lived cultures, relationships are held to be of primary importance, and they are based on trust and mutual well-being. Some, such as the pygmies of Central Africa, have no words for hatred or war, and in their society crime and police do not exist! The Rarámuri (also called Tarahumara) are a group of agrarian runners living in Mexico's Copper Canyon. Held by the running community worldwide to be an example of running purity and excellence, they were featured recently in Christopher McDougall's wildly popular book Born to Run. The Raramuri habitually run for miles on rocky trails in huaraches made of thin leather straps and rubber tire soles. They hold central a powerful belief they call *korima*, which basically means "share with me." They believe they have the duty – or as they see it, the right - to help each other out. Their *korima* is a far cry from the me centered culture that most may recognize as their own. Here we are reminded of the words of one doctor/author: "Listen with regard when others talk. Give your time and energy to others; let others have their way; do things for reasons other than furthering your own needs."

The type-A driven society of today seems to be at odds with this advice, but at what consequence? It is important to note that men who use the first-person pronouns the most often have the highest risk of heart trouble.

The poet John Donne wrote that no man is an island, and we all know that you cannot live in this world without the support of others. You certainly cannot thrive. Chronic loneliness is one of the most lethal risk factors for premature death, while volunteering at a soup kitchen or hospital has been associated with life extension.

Regular acts of altruism prolong our lives and improve our own happiness. Being kind to others reduces stress, bolsters immunity, and provides a sense of joy, peace, and well-being, even relief from physical and emotional pain.

Being involved in some social network - whether it is family, friends, church, volunteer groups, or marriage – adds to your years. In fact, there is evidence to suggest that maintaining close social ties can effectively cancel out some harmful lifestyle choices, such as smoking, obesity, and lack of exercise, and prolong the life of a social junk-food eater beyond that of the exercising health-food eating loner. And if you're not a people person, pets work just as well.

Touching is an essential part of human nurturing from birth onward and results in the release of several feel-good chemicals in the brain, as well as altered gene expression. This is because the semiconductive properties of the connective tissue are far superior in speed and power to other to other signaling mechanisms. Hence the popular saying attributed to psychotherapist Virginia Satir: "Four hugs a day are necessary for survival, eight are good for maintenance, and twelve for growth."

The American anthropologist Ruth Benedict conducted extensive research on so-called "synergistic" societies and helped elucidate why some cultures are cooperative while others are competitive. Within these societies, behaviors benefitting the whole group are rewarded, while harmful behaviors are forbidden. Because generosity and compassion are esteemed over hoarding and flaunting wealth, money continuously circulates through the community rather than accumulating in the hands of a few individuals. Garden produce, horses, cattle, and other valuable goods give a person no standing unless they benefit the tribe at large. In contrast to the synergistic societies are those that are surly and nasty, those in which selfish behaviors are rewarded, and individuals who amass wealth are esteemed. In these societies, people tend to be paranoid, mean-spirited, and aggressive, and wealth belongs to a small few. If this society sounds too familiar let your kindness be the exception to the rule.

Take-home point: *Be the change you wish to see in the world.*

## 14. Find your flow

Youth is not a time of life but a state of mind. It is characterized by idealism and by enthusiasm.

To live long and fruitfully, you have to want to stick around, and longevity is associated with having a purpose. Something you do not because you have to, not as a means to an end, but because you want to, because the act itself has meaning. The best of both worlds occurs if what you love to do also happens to be how you earn your living. Think of your favorite restaurant chefs, musicians and artists, even UPS delivery persons. Your flow may be in writing poetry, exercising, cuddling your children, or simply washing the dishes, any act that you simultaneously lose yourself in and yet are never more present in the moment than when you are doing it.

While most organs stop growing in our late teens, our brains – with ongoing stimulation, discovery, physical exercise, new environments – can continue to change and be shaped our entire lives. Neurons are wired to respond to novel events, and as long as we fill our life with new experiences, just like exercise produces new capillaries, we keep stimulating neurogenesis, the formation of new neurons. Moreover, since we are building these neural pathways with every thought and feeling, we have an opportunity, by taking control of the quality of our thoughts and feelings, to build a brain that transmits positive, healing, and joyful impulses. Wayne Dyer talks about following your bliss. That pretty much sums it up.

## 15. Keep it simple

Happiness, which like VO2 max and other biomarkers happens to be a measure of longevity, does not increase with the money you earn. Of course, not having enough money can cause distress and shorten life. Worldwide, those nations whose annual per capita income is below about $10,000 often suffer from poor sanitation and malnutrition and have the poorest health. But once your basic needs are met, too much money can be a hindrance in that it overly complicates things. The point beyond which money ceases to contribute to happiness is around $50,000 per year. Above the minimum threshold, health ceases to be about income and is more influenced by the gap between the rich and the poor. In other words, a large gap between rich and poor adversely affects you health.

Consider that the United States, last among industrialized nations in wealth equality, where the gap between the richest one percent and the rest of us is the greatest, also happens to be nearly last in life expectancy. With only about 5 percent of the world's population, the US accounts for nearly 50 percent of the world's spending on healthcare. But despite the tremendous amount of money spent on medicine (in the trillions), we don't even rank in the top 20 in life expectancy. In asociety characterized by the haves and have nots, it is natural to guard your possessions and distrust your neighbors, with a corresponding increase in crime, violence, and, not coincidentally, in heart disease, mental disorders, and other deadly conditions affecting rich and poor alike.

How to become less materialistic and simplify your life? Start by cleaning out your space. If it's not beautiful or practical, question the need for the presence of a particular item. The emphasis should not be on ownership but on utility. What you own ends up owning you, so give superfluities away, and share.

## 16. Log off

The average computer user spends 75 minutes on Facebook and logs in 6 times per day. Is this healthy? No, says the scientific literature. Too much time online – whether in front of the computer or vial your handheld device - can lead to stress, sleeping disorders, and depression. Whether you're working, gaming, or chatting, too much time logged in tends to lead to time pressure, neglect of other activities and personal needs (such as social interaction, sleep, physical activity), as well as bad ergonomics and mental overload.

The dangers of cellphone use are currently being debated in the scientific community. While the National Cancer Institute's website states that studies have not shown a consistent link between cell phone use and cancers, it is recognized that more research is needed, as cell phone technology and cell phone use are continuing to change rapidly. But in other countries, the evidence seems more clear. Consider that in Scotland cell phone towers are not allowed to be located near hospitals, schools, and homes. The documentary "Public Exposure: DNA, Democracy and the Wireless Revolution," provides an excellent look at the connection between radio frequency radiation and human health.

Regular exposure to radio frequency radiation (the kind of radiation emitted by cellular phones) may interfere with the electrical fields of our cells. This may lead to abnormal cell growth and damage to cellular DNA, difficulty sleeping, depression, anxiety, and irritability, leukemia, eye cancer, immunosuppression, attention deficit and memory loss, even infertility. Because of their thinner and smaller skulls, children are at much higher risk than adults of experiencing health problems related to regular exposure to radio frequency radiation. From the early 1950's to the mid 1970's, the U.S. embassy in Moscow was purposefully bombarded by radio frequency radiation 24 hours a day. As a result, the U.S. embassy workers experienced what the perpetrators identified as "Radio Frequency

Sickness Syndrome," characterized by headaches, dizziness, and depression.

Why isn't the public aware of the risks of EM exposure? Simple. According to Dr. Phillips, a biochemist and researcher who once worked for Motorola, the only significant money available to do research on cell phone safety issues is industry money, and industry power to suppress unfavorable results is formidable.

Despite "unclear evidence," the National Cancer Institute recommends reserving the use of cell phones for shorter conversations or for times when a landline phone is not available, and using a hands-free device, which places more distance between the phone and the head of the user in order to minimize radiofrequency radiation. A simple device - called a Gauss meter - can help you discover any EMF "hot spots" that might exist in your living and work areas.

Take-home point: *Set limits on the time you spend in front of a screen or on the phone, and limit demands on your availability to avoid stress and mental disorders, which can shorten lifespan and make the years you do have seem miserable.*

## 17. Be positive

Norman Shealy has described four personality types linked to longevity. The first type is characterize by hopelessness, the second by blame and anger, the third by hopelessness and anger; the fourth personality type is self-actualized, believing happiness is an inside job. People in the fourth category tend to die of old age (are the longest lived) rather than of cancer or heart disease.

The importance of maintaining a positive outlook cannot be stressed enough. A host of exciting research has shown how much attitude affects our health. In a widely-cited study, people who had positive perceptions of aging lived an average of 7.5 years longer than those with negative images of growing older. In another study, this one of heart patients, people with positive attitudes who exercised had a 42 percent decreased chance of dying over the study period, while 16.5 percent of those with more negative attitudes died. Having a cheerful disposition lowers heart attack risk, and positive thinking about the future is linked with a lower risk of dying from heart disease. It is important to remember that heart disease is America's number one killer. The antidote to the most common cause of death therefore seems to be a bright attitude.

Being psychologically young involves having a positive mental attitude, staying cognitively and physically active, and having a high-quality life. Optimists are less likely to become frail, defined as impaired strength or endurance, balance problems, and vulnerability to trauma and other stresses, than the pessimists of the bunch.

According to a Mayo Clinic study . . . but do we really need more evidence? It is resoundingly clear that attitude is of paramount importance, that thinking positively can influence your longevity and other health parameters perhaps more than any other factor.

Take-home point: *Like the blood type, be positive.*

## 18. Don't retire, and don't rush.

Longevity is associated with regular work, especially in a relaxed environment without deadlines.

The scientific literature has consistently shown a correlation between early retirement and earlier death. In fact, for every extra year of early retirement, you can expect to lose about two months of life expectancy. Work, whether paid or volunteer, is in part what keeps people living to advanced ages. If your full-time career is too taxing, consider working part-time, switching to a less stressful job, or volunteering.

## 19. De-stress

Hans Selve, the German physician who coined the term "stress" originally broke it down into two types: distress, or negative stress, and eustress, or positive stress – the kind of stress that causes an athlete to excel. Researchers have studied the effects of stress on the immune system and found that during stressful periods production of the molecule interleukin-2 (IL-2), which instructs white blood cells to attack invaders, drops significantly, leading to immune suppression. Conversely, eustress is not associated with a drop in the production of IL-2. Also of note, stresses such as physical traumas and stressful social or psychological situations (interoffice rivalries, marital disagreements, traffic) lead to the production of a protein called Fos, which is also overexpressed in severe forms of cancer and predicts a poor prognosis.

At all times within your body, a tug of war takes place between the chemical mediators cortisol and DHEA. Both are made by your adrenal glands and both share the same chemical precursors, but they have vastly different biochemical and physiological effects. DHEA has health-promoting functions, and is associated with cell repair. The stress hormone cortisol is associated with a host of harmful effects: cortisol sucks resources away from cell repair, kills brain cells, and has been shown to reduce muscle mass, increase bone loss and increase the accumulation of fat around the waist and hips; it also reduces memory and learning abilities. Long-term stress, which keeps brain cortisol levels chronically high, damages the hippocampus, the structure of the brain associated with long-term memory, inhibiting memory and learning.

Being under serious emotional stress, whether the source is financial troubles, job insecurity, legal problems, or marital strife, can more than triple your risk of dying during the next seven years. In fact, your level of stress is a stronger predictor of dying than medical indicators such as high blood pressure and high cholesterol. We cannot escape stressful situations, but there is an antidote. Developing a network of intimate connections – spouse, family members, close friends – can neutralize the harmful effects of life stressors and lowers the production of stress chemicals such as cortisol and catecholamines – provided of course that your loved ones are supportive and not an additional source of woe.

There are many techniques for dealing with stress. One of the easiest is to smile. Even if you don't feel like cracking a grin, just using the muscles active in a smile convinces your body you are happy and sends a surge of feel-good chemicals through your circulation. And if you're really in the mood, add a few hearty laughs. Laughter has been shown to improve mood more than smiling alone.

Meditation, all by itself, may offer more to the health of a modern American than all the pharmaceutical remedies put together. Daily relaxation for just thirty minutes lowers adrenaline production and insulin requirements by 50 percent for twenty-four hours.

The neuroscientist Richard Davidson of the University of Madison at Wisconsin has investigated the areas of the brain that are active during meditation, specifically in Tibetan Buddhist monks. The brain scans of these daily meditators show a higher proportion of gamma waves - the type involved in attention, memory, and learning – and more brain activity in areas linked to positive emotions like happiness. Subjects instructed in Buddhist techniques and who meditated for just thirty minutes a day improved their moods as much as if they had taken antidepressants –

without the negative side effects of prescriptive medication. Meditation is an effective way to bulk up the portions of the brain that produce happiness. And it is not necessary to sit still in order to still the mind. The marathon monks of Mount Hiei cover 52.5 miles per day, equivalent to two marathons, each day over a 100-day stretch as part of a 7-year running program purported to lead to enlightenment.

Take-home point: *Strive to achieve at least thirty minutes daily of deep relaxation through meditation. Avoid negative news, violent movies, excessive television viewing. Think meditation over medication.*

And, perhaps most importantly:

## 20. Be happy

An analysis of several studies conducted by the Dutch professor Ruut Veenhovven found that happiness alone can add between seven and ten years to your lifespan. That's more than not smoking! If you're happy, you're more likely to control your weight, detect the early symptoms of illness, and monitor your alcohol intake and dietary consumption. On the other hand, chronic unhappiness activates the fight or flight response, which if chronically stimulated leads to higher blood pressure and a lower immune response.

What's more, happiness is contagious! Having a friend who is happy increases your chances of happiness by 15%, as shown in a large scale study of residents of Framingham, Massachusetts, from 1983 on. There seems to be truth to the saying: "Smile and the world smiles with you." Why not be that friend to others?

You may not have control over all your life's circumstances, but your reaction to them is within your power, and if you greet each day with exuberance and hope, it is likely to be a self-fulfilling prophesy of fortune.

Take-home point: *To date, no one has managed to defeat death, or for that matter to live past 120 years. And even if you have found the key to longevity, tomorrow you may get run over by a car. (It happened to us, and is the subject of another book.)*

*Finding the fountain of youth is not about living forever, but about living each day like its your last, knowing that when tomorrow comes, it will be better for the effort.*

Made in the USA
San Bernardino, CA
11 March 2014